INTRODUCTION

In the battle against lung cancer, no one has to combat the illness alone. That's where the knowledge in this book can be useful. Lung Cancer: Your Questions & Answers provides knowledgeable and helpful responses to the most frequently asked questions by patients and their families. What is NSCLC, or non-small cell lung cancer? What leads to lung cancer? How is the treatment for lung cancer?

This book includes several new appendices with useful information, including staging criteria for non-small cell lung cancer, crucial questions to ask your doctor, and a complete list of sites for more information. Lung Cancer: Your Questions and Answers is a priceless tool for anyone managing the psychological and physical uncertainty associated with this illness.

DISCLAIMER

This decision aid's content is solely intended for general health information. Only the answers you enter into the risk calculator will allow it to estimate your risk. We make every effort to present the most accurate estimates we can, but for a given individual, the statistics might not be correct. Certain risk variables might exist that are not quantified. As a result, you should never use the material on this website in place of professional medical advice. Please discuss your concerns with your physician or other healthcare practitioner if you have any worries about lung cancer or your chance of developing it.

Table of Contents

1

WHAT IS LUNG CANCER?

An illness known as cancer occurs when body cells proliferate uncontrollably. Lung cancer is the term for cancer that originates in the lungs.

Lung cancer starts in the lungs and can go to other organs including the brain or lymph nodes. Lung cancer can potentially spread from other organs. We refer to the spread of cancer cells from one organ to another as metastases.

Small cell and non-small cell lung cancers are the two primary categories into which lung cancers are typically classified (non-small cell includes adenocarcinoma and squamous cell carcinoma). These variations in lung cancer growth and treatment are noted. Compared to small cell lung cancer, non-small cell lung cancer occurs more frequently.

Furthermore, unchecked cell growth is the cause of lung cancer.

Cancer is a disease in which cells in the body grow out of control. When cancer starts in the lungs, it is called lung cancer.

Lung cancer begins in the lungs and may spread to lymph nodes or other organs in the body, such as the brain. Cancer from other organs also may spread to the lungs. When cancer cells spread from one organ to another, they are called metastases.

Lung cancers usually are grouped into two main types called small cell and non-small cell (non-small cell includes adenocarcinoma and squamous cell carcinoma). These types of lung cancer grow differently and are treated differently. Non-small cell lung cancer is more common than small cell lung cancer.

Furthermore,Lung cancer is a disease caused by uncontrolled cell division in your lungs. Your cells divide and make more copies of themselves as a part of their normal function. But sometimes, they get changes (mutations) that cause them to keep making more of themselves when they shouldn't. Damaged cells dividing uncontrollably create masses, or tumors, of tissue that eventually keep your organs from working properly.

Lung cancer is the name for cancers that start in your lungs — usually in the airways (bronchi or bronchioles) or small air sacs (alveoli). Cancers that start in other places and move to your lungs are usually named for where they start (your healthcare provider may refer to this as cancer that's metastatic to your lungs).

3

EARLY SIGNS OF LUNG CANCER

What are the Signs of lung cancer?

Most lung cancer symptoms look similar to other, less serious illnesses. Many people don't have symptoms until the disease is advanced, but some people have symptoms in the early stages. For those who do experience symptoms, it may only be one or a few of these:

- A cough that doesn't go away or gets worse over time.

- Trouble breathing or shortness of breath (dyspnea).

- Chest pain or discomfort.

- Wheezing.

- Coughing up blood (hemoptysis).

- Hoarseness.

- Loss of appetite.

- Unexplained weight loss.

- Unexplained fatigue (tiredness).

- Shoulder pain.

- Swelling in the face, neck, arms or upper chest (superior vena cava syndrome).

- Small pupil and drooping eyelid in one eye with little or no sweating on that side of your face (Horner's syndrome).

4

STAGES OF LUNG CANCER

Cancer is usually staged based on the size of the initial tumor, how far or deep into the surrounding tissue it goes, and whether it's spread to lymph nodes or other organs. Each type of cancer has its own guidelines for staging.

Lung cancer staging

Each stage has several combinations of size and spread that can fall into that category. For instance, the primary tumor in a Stage III cancer could be smaller than in a Stage II cancer, but other factors put it at a more advanced stage. The general staging for lung cancer is:

Stage 0 (in-situ): Cancer is in the top lining of the lung or bronchus. It hasn't spread to other parts of the lung or outside of the lung.

Stage I: Cancer hasn't spread outside the lung.

Stage II: Cancer is larger than Stage I, has spread to lymph nodes inside the lung, or there's more than one tumor in the same lobe of the lung.

Stage III: Cancer is larger than Stage II, has spread to nearby lymph nodes or structures or there's more than one tumor in a different lobe of the same lung.

Stage IV: Cancer has spread to the other lung, the

fluid around the lung, the fluid around the heart or distant organs.

Limited vs. extensive stage

While providers now use stages I through IV for small cell lung cancer, you might also hear it described as limited or extensive stage. This is based on whether the area can be treated with a single radiation field.

Limited stage SCLC is confined to one lung and can sometimes be in the lymph nodes in the middle of the chest or above the collar bone on the same side.

Extensive stage SCLC is widespread throughout one lung or has spread to the other lung, lymph nodes on the opposite side of the lung, or to other parts of the body.

What is metastatic lung cancer?

Metastatic lung cancer is cancer that starts in one lung but spreads to the other lung or to other organs. Metastatic lung cancer is harder to treat than cancer that hasn't spread outside of its original location.

5

HOW IS LUNG CANCER DIAGNOSED

How lung cancer is diagnosed differs from person to

person. Your medical team chooses tests based on several factors:

Your medical history

Your symptoms

Findings from your physical exam and test results

IMAGING TESTS

Your doctor might order imaging tests that may help find lung cancer. Imaging tests make pictures of the inside of your body. These pictures help doctors to find lung cancer, to see if it has spread, to see if treatment is working or to find a cancer that has come back after treatment. These tests include:

Computed tomography (CT) scan

A CT (or CAT) scan is a special kind of x-ray that takes many pictures as you lie on a table that slides in and out of the machine. A computer then combines these pictures into a detailed picture of a slice of your body.

Positron emission tomography (PET) scan

For a PET scan, a form of radioactive sugar isotope is injected into the blood. Cancer cells in the body absorb large amounts of the sugar. A special camera can then detect the radioactivity. This test can helps determine whether the cancer has spread to the lymph nodes or other parts of the body.

Procedures

To see if something suspicious is actually lung cancer, the doctor must study tissue or fluid from or around the lung. Many different procedures allow doctors to remove cells or biopsy from the body and look at them under a microscope to determine if they are cancer. These tests include:

Bronchoscopy biopsy

A lighted, flexible tube (called a bronchoscope) is passed through the mouth or nose and into the large airways of the lungs. This test can help the doctor see tumors, or it can be used to take samples of tissue to see if cancer cells are present.

Endobronchial ultrasound (EBUS)

For endobronchial ultrasound, a bronchoscope (a thin, lighted, flexible tube) is fitted with an ultrasound device (a device that uses sound waves to make pictures of the inside of your body) at its tip. It is passed down into the windpipe to look at nearby lymph nodes and other structures in the chest. This is done with numbing medicine (local anesthesia) and sedation. A hollow needle can be passed through the bronchoscope and guided by ultrasound into an area of concern to take biopsy samples.

Endoscopic esophageal ultrasound (EUS)

This test is much like an endobronchial ultrasound, except that an endoscope (a lighted, flexible tube) is used. It is passed down the throat and into the esophagus and used as a guide to evaluate and sample adjacent lymph nodes.

Mediastinoscopy and mediastinotomy

Both of these tests let the surgeon look at and take samples of lymph nodes in the area between the lungs (this area is called the mediastinum).

Thoracentesis

This test is done to check whether fluid around the lungs is caused by cancer or by some other medical problem. A needle is placed between the ribs to drain the fluid. The fluid is checked for cancer cells.

Thoracoscopy or video-assisted thoracoscopic surgery (VATS) biopsy

A small cut is made in the chest. The surgeon then uses a thin, lighted tube connected to a video camera and screen to look at the space between the lungs and the chest wall. The surgeon can see small tumors on the lung or lining of the chest wall and can take out pieces of tissue to be looked at under the microscope. Thoracoscopy can also be used as part of the treatment to remove part of a lung in some early-stage lung cancers. Video-assisted thoracic surgery (VATS) is a new type of surgery that allows surgeons to make very small incisions to view the inside of the chest cavity and potentially remove the cancer.

Sputum cytology

A sample of mucus you cough up from the lungs (called sputum or phlegm) is examined under a microscope to see if cancer cells are present.

Fine needle aspiration (FNA) biopsy

A long, thin (fine) needle is used to remove a sample of cells from the area that may be cancer. The sample is examined in the lab to see if it contains cancer cells.

Open biopsy

Under general anesthesia an incision is made in the chest, between the ribs, to obtain a tissue sample or to remove the cancer.

Many researchers are working to develop tests that can make a difference in early lung cancer screening and survival. If you think you are at risk for lung cancer or if you have any symptoms, talk to your doctor about tests to see if you have lung cancer.

IS LUNG CANCER CURABLE?

It depends on the stage and type of lung cancer, and each case is unique. However, in general, some types of lung cancer are curable with treatment, while others are not. Early-stage lung cancer, such as stage 1 or 2, is more likely to be curable with treatment, while later-stage lung cancer, such as stage 4, is more difficult to cure. It's best to speak with a doctor to get a personalized prognosis and treatment plan. The good news is that with advances in research and treatment, survival rates for lung cancer are improving.

Absolutely! One thing to keep in mind is that even if lung cancer is not curable, it may still be treatable to slow the progression of the disease and improve quality of life. For example, treatment may help to shrink tumors, relieve symptoms, and improve overall survival. There are a variety of treatments available, including surgery, radiation therapy, chemotherapy, targeted therapy, and immunotherapy. It's important to discuss all of the treatment options with a doctor to find the best course of action.

7

HOW IS LUNG CANCER TREATED?

Treatments for lung cancer are designed to get rid

of cancer in your body or slow down its growth. Treatments can remove cancerous cells, help to destroy them or keep them from multiplying or teach your immune system to fight them. Some therapies are also used to reduce symptoms and relieve pain. Your treatment will depend on the type of lung cancer you have, where it is, how far it's spread and many other factors.

What medications/treatments are used in lung cancer?

Lung cancer treatments include surgery, radiofrequency ablation, radiation therapy, chemotherapy, targeted drug therapy and immunotherapy.

Surgery

NSCLC that hasn't spread and SCLC that's limited to a single tumor can be eligible for surgery. Your surgeon might remove the tumor and a small amount of healthy tissue around it to make sure they don't leave any cancer cells behind. Sometimes they have to remove all or part of your lung (resection) for the best chance that the cancer won't come back.

Radiofrequency ablation

NSCLC tumors near the outer edges of your lungs are sometimes treated with radiofrequency ablation (RFA). RFA uses high-energy radio waves to heat and destroy cancer cells.

Radiation therapy

Radiation uses high energy beams to kill cancer cells. It can be used by itself or to help make surgery more effective. Radiation can also be used as palliative care, to shrink tumors and relieve pain. It's used in both NSCLC and SCLC.

Chemotherapy

Chemotherapy is often a combination of multiple medications designed to stop cancer cells from growing. It can be given before or after surgery or in combination with other types of medication, like immunotherapy. Chemotherapy for lung cancer is usually given through an IV.

Targeted drug therapy

In some people with NSCLC, lung cancer cells have

specific changes (mutations) that help the cancer grow. Special drugs target these mutations to try to slow down or destroy cancer cells. Other drugs, called angiogenesis inhibitors, can keep the tumor from creating new blood vessels, which the cancer cells need to grow.

Immunotherapy

Our bodies usually recognize cells that are damaged or harmful and destroy them. Cancer has ways to hide from the immune system to keep from being destroyed. Immunotherapy reveals cancer cells to your immune system so your own body can fight cancer.

Treatments to ease symptoms (palliative care)

Some lung cancer treatments are used to relieve symptoms, like pain and difficulty breathing. These include therapies to reduce or remove tumors that are blocking airways, and procedures to remove fluid from around your lungs and keep it from coming back.

8

WHAT TREATMENT RELATED SIDE EFFECTS SHOULD I EXPECT?

Side effects of the treatment

Side effects of lung cancer treatment depend on the type of treatment. Your provider can tell you what side effects to expect, and what complications to look out for, for your specific treatment.

Chemotherapy

Nausea, vomiting.

Diarrhea.

Hair loss.

Fatigue.

Mouth sores.

Loss of feeling, weakness or tingling (neuropathy).

Immunotherapy

Fatigue.

Itchy rash.

Diarrhea.

Nausea, vomiting.

Joint pain.

Complications (like pneumonitis, colitis, hepatitis and others) can have additional side effects.

Radiation therapy

Shortness of breath.

Cough.

Pain.

Fatigue.

Difficulty swallowing.

Dry, itchy or red skin.

Nausea, vomiting.

Surgery

Shortness of breath.

Chest wall pain.

Cough.

Fatigue.

How do I manage symptoms and side effects?

Your provider can prescribe medications to help manage your symptoms or side effects of treatment. A palliative care specialist or a dietitian can help you manage pain or other symptoms and improve your quality of life while you're in treatment.

9

IS LUNG CANCER ASSOCIATED WITH SMOKING?

Cigarette smoking is the number one risk factor for lung cancer. In the United States, cigarette smoking is linked to about 80% to 90% of lung cancer deaths. Using other tobacco products such as cigars or pipes also increases the risk for lung cancer. Tobacco smoke is a toxic mix of more than 7,000 chemicals. Many are poisons. At least 70 are known to cause cancer in people or animals.

People who smoke cigarettes are 15 to 30 times more likely to get lung cancer or die from lung cancer than people who do not smoke. Even smoking a few cigarettes a day or smoking occasionally increases the risk of lung cancer. The more years a person smokes and the more cigarettes smoked each day, the more risk goes up.

People who quit smoking have a lower risk of lung cancer than if they had continued to smoke, but their risk is higher than the risk for people who never smoked. Quitting smoking at any age can lower the risk of lung cancer.

Cigarette smoking can cause cancer almost anywhere in the body. Cigarette smoking causes cancer of the mouth and throat, esophagus, stomach, colon, rectum, liver, pancreas, voicebox (larynx), lung, trachea, bronchus, kidney and renal pelvis, urinary bladder, and cervix, and causes acute myeloid leukemia.

Secondhand Smoke

Smoke from other people's cigarettes, pipes, or cigars (secondhand smoke) also causes lung cancer. In the United States, one out of four people who don't smoke, including 14 million children, were exposed to secondhand smoke during 2013 to 2014.

10

HOW DO I REDUCE THE RISK OF LUNG

There's no sure way to prevent lung cancer, but you can reduce your risk if you:

Don't smoke. **If you've never smoked, don't start. Talk to your children about not smoking so that they can understand how to avoid this major risk factor for lung cancer. Begin conversations about the dangers of smoking with your children early so that they know how to react to peer pressure.**

Stop smoking. **Stop smoking now. Quitting reduces your risk of lung cancer, even if you've smoked for years. Talk to your doctor about strategies and stop-smoking aids that can help you quit. Options include nicotine replacement products, medications and** support groups.

Avoid secondhand smoke. **If you live or work with a smoker, urge him or her to quit. At the very least, ask him or her to smoke outside. Avoid areas where people smoke, such as bars and restaurants, and seek out smoke-free options.**

Test your home for radon. **Have the radon levels in your home checked, especially if you live in an area where radon is known to be a problem. High radon levels can be remedied to make your home safer. For information on radon testing, contact your local department of public health or a local chapter of the American Lung Association.**

Avoid carcinogens at work. **Take precautions to protect yourself from exposure to toxic chemicals at work. Follow your employer's precautions. For instance, if you're given a face mask for protection,** always wear it. Ask your doctor what more you can do to protect yourself at work. Your risk of lung damage from workplace carcinogens increases if you smoke.

Eat a diet full of fruits and vegetables. Choose a healthy diet with a variety of fruits and vegetables. Food sources of vitamins and nutrients are best. Avoid taking large doses of vitamins in pill form, as they may be harmful. For instance, researchers hoping to reduce the risk of lung cancer in heavy smokers gave them beta carotene supplements. Results showed the supplements actually increased the risk of cancer in smokers.

Exercise most days of the week. If you don't exercise regularly, start out slowly. Try to exercise most days of the week

11

CONCLUSION

Treatment of lung cancer is complex and requires accurate knowledge of both the anatomic stage of the tumor and the patient's overall physiologic condition. Surgical treatment of lung cancer may be an option for patients once thought to be medically unresectable, and patients with borderline physiologic reserve should be seen by a multidisciplinary team. Postoperative adjuvant chemotherapy is now the standard of care for patients with stage II and III non-small cell lung cancer. Therapeutic nihilism for patients who are not candidates for curative surgery should be particularly discouraged; even patients with significant comorbidity can receive curative therapy that preserves quality of life while offering cure or prolonging survival. Patients and clinicians often have an unrealistically pessimistic outlook on the potential benefits of lung cancer treatment. Aggressive multimodality therapy for locally advanced, unresectable (stage III) NSCLC can still offer otherwise healthy patients a significant survival benefit, with 15% to 20% of patients achieving long-term survival. Therefore, patients with clinical stage III NSCLC should be offered realistic but hopeful assessment of their treatment options. Metastatic (stage IV) NSCLC is generally incurable, but also treatable.

Respiratory medicine physicians and other clinicians need to provide cancer patients with the best possible treatment, and in those with metastatic lung cancer and preserved performance status, this includes lung cancer–specific treatment, perhaps alongside early palliative care. Newer treatment options are becoming available at a rapid pace, and the role of novel, targeted therapies is being defined more precisely.

Treatment of lung cancer has evolved dramatically over the past 20 years with a better understanding of underlying genomics. This is the best exemplified in metastatic lung adenocarcinoma where there are now multiple genomic alterations with effective targeted therapy. Immune therapy also has improved outcomes for many patients and ongoing efforts are focused on how genomic alterations interact with the tumor immune microenvironment to develop personalized strategies to optimize therapy. Finally, the use of cfDNA offers hope for more precision detection and prognostication in early stage NSCLC. Advancements in each of these aspects of genomic medicine are eagerly awaited as personalized medicine is expected to continue to improve outcomes for patients with lung cancer.